YOUR KNOWLEDGE HAS VALUE

AF166931

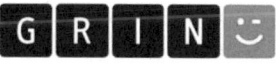

Polymer- and Lipid-Based Cancer Nanotheranostics

Nazli Irmak Giritlioglu
Gizem Köprülülü Küçük

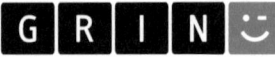

Bibliographic information published by the German National Library:

The German National Library lists this publication in the National Bibliography; detailed bibliographic data are available on the Internet at http://dnb.dnb.de.

ISBN: 9783346205094
This book is also available as an ebook.

Print and binding: Books on Demand GmbH, Norderstedt, Germany
Printed on acid-free paper from responsible sources.

The present work has been carefully prepared. Nevertheless, authors and publishers do not incur liability for the correctness of information, notes, links and advice as well as any printing errors.

GRIN web shop: https://www.hausarbeiten.de/document/903290

POLYMER- AND LIPID- BASED CANCER NANOTHERANOSTICS

TABLE OF CONTENTS

INTRODUCTION

Cancer is a worldwide threat and there is no efficient cure for many types of this disease which is caused by damage to genes that control cell growth and division. The most important definitive feature of cancer is abnormal cell divisions that occur in various parts of the body and can spread to other organs (Nayak KA.& Pal D., 2010). The abnormal cell division suppresses the tissue or organ that it surrounds, preventing the tissue or organ from functioning. Early diagnosis is an important consideration in cancer treatment. It is difficult to diagnose cancer in the early stages with traditional diagnostic methods. Advances in nanotechnology, which is a multidisciplinary science, offers important opportunities in terms of cancer diagnosis and treatment. Cancer-causing factors can be grouped into two groups, roughly genetically and environmentally. Only 1% of cancers are caused by genetic transport. Disorders in some genes acquired by heredity cause cancer especially in childhood. However, disorders in genes such as BRCA1 and BRCA2 can cause cancer in older ages. For example, in women with these mutated genes, the risk of breast cancer has been observed to increase by 80% compared to the normal population (Ephrat PE. & Sharon LL, 2003). The remaining 99% of cancers depend on people's eating habits, working conditions, living environments, natural or artificial radiation to which they are exposed, and carcinogenic chemicals. These are called environmental cancer risk factors.

In cancer treatments, non-invasively real-time monitoring is a very important issue to determine the progress of healing. And the chemicals used in the treatment have cytotoxic properties, but these drugs must only kill the cancer cells. Practically, we can observe the cytotoxic effects on the cells and show drug efficiency. Also, animals are useful models for these kinds of experiments. On the other hand, these drugs kill normal cells too. This is the situation that we don't want to as cancer researchers. The cancer researchers try to improve the platforms with high efficiency for cancer treatment, which don't kill healthy cells, carry the drug to the exact desired point (cancer tissue), and be monitored by the doctors.

In this book; we mention cancer treatment, diagnosis with nanotechnology relations, and polymer and lipid-based (LB) nanotheranostic platforms.

1. Using Nanotechnology in Cancer Diagnosis and Treatment

Cancer is a disease that takes a long time to develop. It provides convenience in the treatment of diagnosis in the early stages. If the cells can be intervened in the early stages of the mutation, cancer development can be stopped (Auyang YS., 2006). In classical methods used in cancer diagnosis, X-Ray and / or CT scans detect growths and changes in organs. In suspicious cases, the diagnosis of cancer is clarified by performing a biopsy. Early diagnosis is not possible with these methods. In most cases, they can be visualized when the tumor reaches a diameter of 1 cm or weight of about 1 g. In this case, the number of cancerous cells is approximately 108. 2/3 of cancer cases were diagnosed when the case became fatal (Wang X. et al., 2004). Various problems encountered in conventional diagnostic methods reduce the efficiency of these methods.

With the help of nanotechnology, tumors can be diagnosed early. The ability of nanostructures to enter a single tumor cell increases the limits of imaging techniques in this regard. For example, in order to make a clinical diagnosis of breast cancer by mammography, 1.000.000 tumor cells must have been formed. With the help of nanotechnology, it is possible to diagnose breast cancer even when less than 100 tumor cells are formed (Singh KK., 2005). For early cancer diagnosis, cancer-specific biomolecules and nanostructures capable of forming bioconjugation are also used.

Radiotherapy, chemotherapy, and surgery are the main methods used in cancer treatment. Surgical methods consist of resection (removal) of cancerous tissue. Disadvantages of these methods are loss of organs, risk of recurrence of cancer, and the inability to apply to all types of cancer. In radiotherapy, cancerous cells are burned in the specific frequency band and with specific intensity radiation. Disadvantages of this method are damage to healthy cells as well as cancerous cells, the radiation distribution is not of equal density to all cancer cells and loss of function in the tissue exposed to radiation. In chemotherapy, it is aimed to kill cancer cells with drugs that have toxic effects and to eliminate the mechanisms that cause cancer cells to divide (Nehru MR. & Singh PO., 2008).

Classical chemotherapy drugs do not act targeted in the body. The drugs used affect cancer cells as well as healthy cells. Also, cancer cells do not reach the required doses for treatment (Wang X., et al., 2009). Chemotherapy weakens the patient's immune system and the patient becomes more susceptible to other diseases. Another problem encountered is the state of MDR (Multi-Drug Resistance) developing against anticancer components. All these important side effects are caused by the fact that chemotherapy drugs do not have a tissue-specific effect. In cancer treatment, chemotherapy drugs need to target tumors as much as possible and have a limited effect on healthy tissues. This issue is also important in terms of increasing the life and quality of the patient. Advances in nano-oncology have brought important innovations in

3

targeted drug delivery (Goel HC. et al., 2009). In this way, the intracellular concentrations of drugs in cancer cells can be increased, while the toxic effects on healthy cells can be minimized.

The term "Theranostics" means combining diagnosis and treatment for a variety of diseases on a single platform. Nanotherapy systems, which combine diagnosis, targeted therapy, and monitoring of treatment response, are defined as theranostic nano-medicine (Sumer B.& Gao J., 2008). Theranostic is the name given to the combination of the treatment agent and the diagnostic method used to define the effect of this agent (Kelkar SS.& Reineke TM., 2011). This diagnosis/treatment hybridization matches target-specific therapy with diagnostic information. This method is especially used in personalized medicine applications. This method makes it possible to classify the diseases according to the molecular phenotype, to observe the biodistribution of the molecule, and to monitor the response to treatment (Lee DY. &Li KC., 2011). Many diagnosis and treatment procedures in nuclear medicine are also included in the scope of theranostic. Iodine-131 (I-131) treatment and scintigraphy, which is the most commonly used diagnosis/treatment method, is the best example of the theranostic practice. By combining diagnosis and treatment on a single platform, cellular phenotypes in each tumor are first characterized and then targeted therapy can be applied. In this way, the effectiveness of treatments can be increased by applying personalized treatments instead of general treatments (Sumer B. & Gao J., 2008). Theranostic platforms can be created by adding chemotherapy drugs to nanoparticles currently used as imaging agents.

2. Polymer-based Cancer Nanotheranostics

Cancer nanotheranostics are the nanoplatforms that provide real-time monitoring non-invasively, desired functions using standard procedures in nanotechnology, controlled encapsulated or linked drug loading/releasing, individualized cancer therapy (Bhojani, Van Dort, Rehemtulla, & Ross, 2010; Chen, Zhang, Zhu, Xie, & Chen, 2017). A conventional nanotheranostic platform has two parts which are diagnostic [magnetic resonance imaging (MRI), single-photon emission computed tomography, ultrasound imaging agents, etc.] and therapeutic agents (chemotherapy, radiation therapy agents, etc.) (Chen et al., 2017). Also, the therapeutic part can act as an imaging agent because of its inherent fluorescence property (Luk & Zhang, 2014) (Figure 1). A polymeric nanotheranostic platform must have stability, targeting ability, and effective biodistribution capabilities (Afshar, 2015).

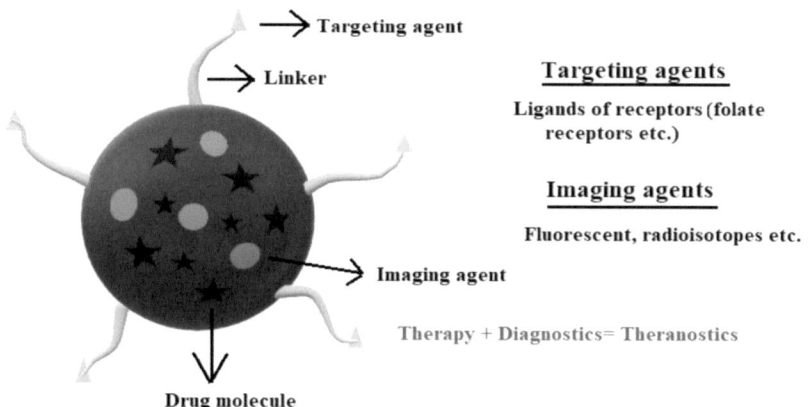

Figure 1. A simple drawing of a nanotheranostic platform.

Any nanotheranostic particle should have three parts: A targeting agent that is generally inside of the particle for targeting the specific location, an imaging agent, and a drug molecule.

The parts of the nanotheranostic platform can be modified by lipids, polymers, and other natural or synthetic structures. Some polymers are preferable to improve the cancer nanotheranostic system because of biocompatibility, versatility, changeable physicochemical properties by adding different functional groups, controllable sizes, and degradation rates (Gopinath, 2015; Sisay, 2014). In the past few decades, the widely thought aim for cancer researchers is to send a cytotoxic agent into the cancerous tissue without sticking to the biological barriers; and in the theranostic area, to monitor the treatment which is using a single nanomedicine. Biological barriers are the main disadvantage of all cancer treatment studies. Successful polymer-, lipid- or any material-based cancer nanotheranostic agents should be prepared to reach exactly into the cancerous target and bypass all barriers on its way. This is one of the important features we call "effectiveness" in cancer treatment. Biological barriers may be separated into two different topics: Immune system, liver, kidneys, blood, spleen, and blood-brain barrier. When a foreign material goes into the body, all these systems cross it with their ways (Kievit & Zhang, 2011).

Reaching the tumor site without structural degradation and not causing an immunogenic effect is a very important issue for any cancer drug after *in vivo* injection. Frank Davis found the idea of PEGylation for a protein in the 1960s (Hoffman, 2016) but nowadays it is a very advantageous way for improving pharmaceutics and Food and Drug Administration (FDA)-

approved PEGylated nanomedicines are commercially selling in the market (Bobo, Robinson, Islam, Thurecht, & Corrie, 2016). PEG is a commonly used polymer for drug modification. Covalent, non-covalent conjunction or coating with PEG (all of them are PEGylation) is a good strategy to target cells and tissues, to enhance the pharmacokinetic profile, to improve physicochemically (such as increasing hydrophilicity) and biocompatibility properties, to decrease immunogenicity, to reduce the rate of glomerular filtration, to prolong the blood circulation of the drug half-life in the body. (Kim, Lee, & Chen, 2013; P. Mishra, Nayak, & Dey, 2016; Suk, Xu, Kim, Hanes, & Ensign, 2016; Vllasaliu, Fowler, & Stolnik, 2014). Also, PEG coating can be resistant to aggregation, opsonization, and phagocytosis (Suk et al., 2016) that are all of the unwanted conditions. PEGylation is adaptable for both passive, active, and stimuli-responsive targeting (P. Mishra et al., 2016). 2000, 3400, 5000, 10.000, and 20.000 Da molecular weights of PEG are common in some reported studies (Jokerst, Lobovkina, Zare, & Gambhir, 2011).

PEGylated nanotheranostic studies are in progress. Palao-Suay et al. generated a multifunctional nanopolymeric nanotheranostic system that has three compounds: IR-780 dye, a methacrylic derivate of α-tocopheryl succinate, and the block copolymers of PEG$_{8000}$. They evaluated the cellular uptake, anticancer, and phototherapeutic activities of their synthesized system *in vitro* using breast carcinoma cells (MDA-MB-453) (Palao-Suay et al., 2017). Sun et al. used black phosphorous to design the PEGylated nanotheranostic platform by using a one-pot solventless preparation technique. This biocompatible, water-soluble and photostable nanomedicine which utilizes enhanced permeability and retention (EPR) effect allows photoacoustic imaging and photothermal therapy which turns NIR to heat energy (Sun et al., 2016). Lin et al. designed and synthesized nanotheranostic nanocomplexes with small particle size (<150 nm) have a hydrophilic core (iron oxide and IR780 dye) and hydrophobic shell (PEG and human serum albumin), for ideal cancer photothermal therapy and magnetic resonance imaging (Lin, Huang, Liao, Chuang, & Chang, 2018). Iron oxide nanoparticles (NPs) are commonly seen in the theranostic researches because of its superparamagnetic and acceptable biocompatibility features (Muthu, Leong, Mei, & Feng, 2014). Song et al. found a solution for radioresistance with their synthesized Indium-111-labelled Epidermal Growth Factor (EGF)-Gold-PEG NPs target EGF receptor-positive cancer cells (MDA-MB-468). >%11 of radioactivity and reducing liver uptake were observed (Song, Able, Johnson, & Vallis, 2017).

As much as PEGylation is a successful improvement for pharmaceutical modification, but adverse effects can not be ignored. Hypersensitivity reaction and anaphylactic shock may be

6

occurred caused by PEG (intravenous or oral administration) or its side products (Kolate et al., 2014). Another important problem is the toxicity. Low molecular weight PEG can be acceptable as a nearly non-toxic polymer and toxicity of PEGylated drugs doesn't come up due to PEG toxicity, the toxic part is the most of drug active site itself (Ivens et al., 2015; Liu et al., 2017). Also, it must considerable problem is cellular vacuolation. ≥ 30 kDa molecular weight PEG can cause vacuolation mainly occurs in phagocytes but any change effects on organ function did not be observed (Ivens et al., 2015). Because of PEG immunogenicity and bioaccumulation problems, researchers have investigated the alternatives to PEGylation, such as bonding to carbohydrate polymers (e.g. dextran, hydroxyethyl starch, polysialic acid, and hyaluronic acid), N- and O-glycosylation or lipidation techniques (van Witteloostuijn, Pedersen, & Jensen, 2016).

It was mentioned that also natural polymers such as hyaluronic acid (HA) can be utilized for the cancer nanotheranostics. HA is a natural linear polysaccharide that has the repeating units of N-acetyl-D-glucosamine and D-glucuronic acid. HA is seen in the extracellular matrix of connecting tissues in the body naturally and because of its biocompatible, non-toxic, biodegradable properties, and it is used in the different pharmaceutical areas. (Tripodo et al., 2015). HA-based nanotheranostic systems are investigated. Yang et. al. designed and synthesized a multifunctional theranostic agent to determine the tumor size and location and effective photothermal treatment with real-time monitoring. There are four parts used in this nanotheranostic system: HA, bovine serum albumin, CulnS$_2$-ZnS quantum dots, and magnetic Prussian blue. Effective ablation of tumor *in vivo* nude mice upon NIR light irradiation and more than 89.95 % tumor growth inhibition was seen (Yang et al., 2017). Another study about the HA-based cancer nanotheranostic system was generated by Dubey and Dubey's group. Gemcitabine was used as a chemotherapy drug and dual nuclear imaging (single-photon emission computed tomography/computed tomography) was utilized in this study which has great targeting, imaging, and killing potentials for CD44-overexpressing cells *in vivo* (Dubey et al., 2017).

Chitosan; naturally occurring, second most abundant after cellulose, biocompatible, biodegradable, non-toxic, carbohydrate polymer used in nanotheranostics, is very utilizing in the different biomedical applications such as tissue engineering, medicine, and other biotechnological aims (Ahsan et al., 2018; Ali & Ahmed, 2018; Bharathiraja et al., 2018). In addition to the advantages of chitosan, there are some disadvantages: Low solubility in biological fluids, insolubility in most organic solvents that limits to encapsulation and delivery of hydrophobic drugs. But synthesized chitosan derivatives and modifications of chitosan could improve these disadvantages (Ahsan et al., 2018). Bharathiraja et al. designed and synthesized the chitosan oligosaccharide coated nanotheranostic system functionalized with arginine-glycine-aspartic acid peptide to bind alpha V beta 3 integrins on the cancer cell surface and including palladium for photothermal therapy and photoacoustic imaging (Bharathiraja et al., 2018). Kanval et al. developed a nanoformulation for optical imaging and chemotherapy based on quaternary ammonium palmitoyl glycol chitosan carrier for doxorubicin has fluorescence property itself. Passive targeting to the tumor site was aimed in this study (Kanwal et al., 2019).

Other polymers can also be used in cancer nanotheranostics. Ferber et. al designed two systems to form polymeric nanotheranostic complex based on *N*-(2-hydroxypropyl) methacrylamide (HPMA) copolymer which has water-soluble and non-toxic properties. For the diagnostics, they used self-quenched fluorescent dye Cy5 (SQ-Cy5) reporter prob and paclitaxel for the therapy. Releasing the drug by a simultaneous fluorescent signal depends on the enzymatic degradation of the extracellular matrix in cathepsin B-overexpressing breast cancer cells in this polymeric nanocarrier (Ferber et al., 2014). Lie et al. designed a single multifunctional nanotheranostics system with multimodal imaging and drug delivery functions to solve the BBB problem in the brain metastasis of breast cancer. Their synthesized system is based on poly(methacrylic acid)-polysorbate 80-grafted-starch terpolymer. The multiple contrast agents (Magnetic Resonance contrast agent gadolinium and near-infrared fluorescence probe HF750) and the cationic drug Doxorubicin (Dox) were used in this system. Results from the comparison of the Dox-loaded system and free-Dox control were promising to owe to detect a large number of apoptotic cells in the Dox-loaded system to treat the brain metastasis (Li et al., 2014). Hou et al. designed a multifunctional nanotheranostic system for photoacoustic imaging and photothermal/photodynamic therapy. They synthesized Cu-Sb-S NP around 24 nm and added poly(vinylpyrrolidone) (PVP) for functionalization. It was seen high cell viability values *in vitro*, so it shows that PVP-Cu-Sb-S NPs have a property of biocompatibility. Also, the exhibition of broad Near Infrared (NIR) absorbance and relatively high photothermal conversion efficiency (53.16%), thermal stability, and reactive oxygen species generation effect were observed (Hou et al., 2018).

3. LB Cancer Nanotheranostics

LB nanotheranostics is highly studied and used in different areas, such as atherosclerosis (Nie et al., 2015), infection (Gao, Thamphiwatana, Angsantikul, & Zhang, 2014), rheumatoid arthritis (Albuquerque, Moura, Sarmento, & Reis, 2015) and especially in cancer research (Knights-Mitchell & Romanowski, 2018; Xiong, Nirupama, Sirsi, Lacko, & Hoyt, 2017). LB NPs have biocompatibility and biodegradable features and allow the different modifications and often utilize the EPR effect and accumulate in the tumors due to highly permeable blood vessels (Miller, 2013; Tang, Tang, & Li, 2018). First-generation LB NPs are liposomes and FDA approved 15 liposomal drugs since 1995. (Tang et al., 2018). Liposomes have spherical structure and its unique, water-soluble form that improves the pharmacokinetic properties, can encapsulate hydrophilic agents, so they are protected from degradation and the hydrophobic agents be held into the lipid bilayer (Mulder, Strijkers, van Tilborg, Griffioen, & Nicolay, 2006; Xing, Hwang, & Lu, 2016). An example of liposome-based nanotheranostics, Seleci et al. generated hydrophilic topotecan loaded liposome-hydrophobic CdSe/ZnS quantum dot (QD) theranostic system. They used thin-film hydration and pH-gradient methods for the encapsulation of topotecan and QD (Seleci, Ag Seleci, Scheper, & Stahl, 2017). Liposomes have several disadvantages such as short half-life, poor stability, low solubility and low encapsulation efficiency, immunogenic effects caused by liposomal constituents etc. (Bodke, 2017; Naseri, Valizadeh, & Zakeri-Milani, 2015).

Solid lipid NPs which are 50-1000 nm structures and the alternative carriers to traditional systems such as emulsions, liposomes, and polymeric micro- and NPs since 1991 (Ekambaram, 2012). Compared to polymeric NPs and the liposomes, solid lipid NPs are less toxic, are more available for both hydrophobic and hydrophilic drugs, let managed easily in large-scale production, have the possibility of lyophilization, better storage capability than the liposomes, and synthesis of polymeric NPs need organic solvents (Gopinath, 2015; Kaur, Bhandari, Bhandari, & Kakkar, 2008; Valetti, Mura, Stella, & Couvreur, 2013). Easily get metabolize in the body, to protect from chemical degradation, to provide controlled drug release and drug targeting, and not have toxicity problems are other advantages of solid lipid NPs (Baek & Cho, 2015). Synthesis of solid lipid NPs usually require solid lipids such as fatty acid, partial triglycerides, triglycerides, waxes; emulsifier, and water (Gopinath, 2015). Solid lipid NPs can be prepared by different techniques such as high-pressure homogenization, ultrasonication/high-speed homogenization, solvent evaporation, solvent emulsification-diffusion, supercritical fluid, microemulsion based, spray drying, double emulsion, precipitation, film-ultrasound dispersion methods (Ekambaram, 2012). Matrix type and drug location in the formulation of solid lipid NP determine the release of the drug (V. Mishra et al., 2018). Cellular uptake of solid lipid NPs is dependent on the melting point of the lipid and lipid composition. The melting point of the lipid and uptake efficiency have reverse correlation, uptake efficiency is higher while the melting point is lower (Gopinath, 2015). Kuang et al. designed a containing solid lipid NP theranostic system for photothermal therapy with NIR imaging. It has been provided conjunction of c(RGDyK)-IR780 solid lipid NP for targeting to cells overexpressing $\alpha_v\beta_3$ integrin (Kuang et al., 2017).

Lipids and proteins together can be used in the nanotheranostic area by utilizing biomimetic science. For example, high-density lipoprotein (HDL) or commonly known "good cholesterol" is natural, 8-12 nm diameter nanoparticle have biocompatible, biodegradable, non-toxic, non-immunogenic properties and it is very promising in the drug delivery systems (X. Ma, Song, & Gao, 2018). Many therapeutics such as nucleic acids and drugs can be loaded into HDL or HDL can be used as an imaging agent with some modifications (Thaxton, Rink, Naha, & Cormode, 2016). HDL has apolipoprotein A-1 (Apo A-1) in its structure and Apo A-1 is a ligand for the Scavenger Receptor Class B Type I (SR-B1). SR-B1 is overexpressed in some tumors such as prostate, breast, ovarian, colorectal, pancreatic cancers, and related to proliferation and metastasis (Mooberry, Sabnis, Panchoo, Nagarajan, & Lacko, 2016; Raut et al., 2018). Less invasive approaches with reconstituted HDL became the new cancer treatment way. For example, Xiong et al. generated a high-density lipoprotein-based nanotheranostic system with non-invasive ultrasound (US) therapy. US therapy is a common, safe, and reversible method to get permeable to tumor vessel walls, so any agent can pass through easily. They used IR-780 dye loaded reconstituted high-density lipoprotein NPs for breast cancer treatment. The results were promising and the system could use instead of invasive surgery soon (Xiong et al., 2017).

Also, lipids and polymers together can be used in the cancer nanotheranostics. PEGylation approach is convenient for lipid-based theranostics. Ma et al. generated a biodegradable, phospholipid-PEG based system with dual-modal imaging for photothermal cancer therapy. Indocyanine green was used for fluorescence imaging and SPIO NPs for the magnetic resonance imaging. Results from the study confirmed that tumor targeting and photothermal therapy properties of the NP was effective (Y. Ma, Tong, Bao, Gao, & Dai, 2013). Banerjee et al. studied on designing paclitaxel-loaded solid lipid NPs modified with Tyr-3-octreotide (TOC). This nanotheranostic system containing TOC-PEG-lipid was planned for to inhibit the angiogenic effects and to target somatostatin receptor 2 overexpressing cells for the glioma treatment (Banerjee et al., 2016). Another example, Wang et al. utilized lipid-polyaniline complex for photothermal and antiangiogenic cancer therapy (Wang et al., 2016).

REFERENCES

Afshar, M. A. A., Moloudi, K., Amirrashedi, M., Rashidi, M., Ranjbar, H. S. . (2015). A BRIEF REVIEW ON POLYMER AND PROTEIN BASED NANOTHERANOSTICS *International Journal of Biology, Pharmacy and Allied Sciences, 5 (1)*, 112-128.

Ahsan, S. M., Thomas, M., Reddy, K. K., Sooraparaju, S. G., Asthana, A., & Bhatnagar, I. (2018). Chitosan as biomaterial in drug delivery and tissue engineering. *Int J Biol Macromol, 110*, 97-109. doi:10.1016/j.ijbiomac.2017.08.140

Albuquerque, J., Moura, C. C., Sarmento, B., & Reis, S. (2015). Solid Lipid Nanoparticles: A Potential Multifunctional Approach towards Rheumatoid Arthritis Theranostics. *Molecules, 20*(6), 11103-11118. doi:10.3390/molecules200611103

Ali, A., & Ahmed, S. (2018). A review on chitosan and its nanocomposites in drug delivery. *International Journal of Biological Macromolecules, 109*, 273-286. doi:https://doi.org/10.1016/j.ijbiomac.2017.12.078

Auyang, Y. S. (2006) Cancer Causes and Cancer Research on Many Levels of Complexity, http://www.creatingtechnology.org/biomed/

Baek, J.-S., & Cho, C.-W. (2015). Controlled release and reversal of multidrug resistance by co-encapsulation of paclitaxel and verapamil in solid lipid nanoparticles. *International journal of pharmaceutics, 478*(2), 617-624. doi:10.1016/j.ijpharm.2014.12.018

Banerjee, I., De, K., Mukherjee, D., Dey, G., Chattopadhyay, S., Mukherjee, M., . . . Misra, M. (2016). Paclitaxel-loaded solid lipid nanoparticles modified with Tyr-3-octreotide for enhanced anti-angiogenic and anti-glioma therapy. *Acta Biomater, 38*, 69-81. doi:10.1016/j.actbio.2016.04.026

Bharathiraja, S., Bui, N. Q., Manivasagan, P., Moorthy, M. S., Mondal, S., Seo, H., . . . Oh, J. (2018). Multimodal tumor-homing chitosan oligosaccharide-coated biocompatible palladium nanoparticles for photo-based imaging and therapy. *Sci Rep, 8*(1), 500. doi:10.1038/s41598-017-18966-8

Bhojani, M. S., Van Dort, M., Rehemtulla, A., & Ross, B. D. (2010). Targeted imaging and therapy of brain cancer using theranostic nanoparticles. *Mol Pharm, 7*(6), 1921-1929. doi:10.1021/mp100298r

Bobo, D., Robinson, K. J., Islam, J., Thurecht, K. J., & Corrie, S. R. (2016). Nanoparticle-Based Medicines: A Review of FDA-Approved Materials and Clinical Trials to Date. *Pharm Res, 33*(10), 2373-2387. doi:10.1007/s11095-016-1958-5

Bodke, A. R., Aher, S. S., Saudagar, RB. (2017). A Review on Liposomes *International Journal ofPharma And Chemical Research, 3*(2), 120-127.

Chen, H., Zhang, W., Zhu, G., Xie, J., & Chen, X. (2017). Rethinking cancer nanotheranostics. *Nat Rev Mater, 2*. doi:10.1038/natrevmats.2017.24

Dubey, R. D., Klippstein, R., Wang, J. T.-W., Hodgins, N., Mei, K.-C., Sosabowski, J., . . . Al-Jamal, K. T. (2017). Novel Hyaluronic Acid Conjugates for Dual Nuclear Imaging and Therapy in CD44-Expressing Tumors in Mice In Vivo. *Nanotheranostics, 1*(1), 59-79. doi:10.7150/ntno.17896

Ekambaram, P., Sathali, A. H. A, Priyanka, K. . (2012). SOLID LIPID NANOPARTICLES: A REVIEW. *Scientific Reviews & Communications, 2*(1), 80-102.

Ferber, S., Baabur-Cohen, H., Blau, R., Epshtein, Y., Kisin-Finfer, E., Redy, O., . . . Satchi-Fainaro, R. (2014). Polymeric nanotheranostics for real-time non-invasive optical imaging of breast cancer progression and drug release. *Cancer Lett, 352*(1), 81-89. doi:10.1016/j.canlet.2014.02.022

Gao, W., Thamphiwatana, S., Angsantikul, P., & Zhang, L. (2014). Nanoparticle approaches against bacterial infections. *6*(6), 532-547. doi:doi:10.1002/wnan.1282

Goel, H. C., Kumar, B. , Yadav, P. R. , Moshahid, M. , Rizvi, A. (2009) Recent Developments in Cancer Therapy by Use of Nanotechnology , Digest J Nanomater Biostr. , 4 (1) , 1 – 12.

Gopinath, P., Uday Kumar, S., Matai, I., Bhushan, B., Malwal, D., Sachdev, A., Dubey, P. (2015). *Cancer Nanotheranostics*: Springer Singapore.

Hoffman, A. S. (2016). The early days of PEG and PEGylation (1970s–1990s). *Acta Biomater, 40*, 1-5. doi:https://doi.org/10.1016/j.actbio.2016.05.029

Hou, M., Yan, C., Chen, Z., Zhao, Q., Yuan, M., Xu, Y., & Zhao, B. (2018). Multifunctional NIR-responsive poly(vinylpyrrolidone)-Cu-Sb-S nanotheranostic agent for photoacoustic imaging and photothermal/photodynamic therapy. *Acta Biomater, 74*, 334-343. doi:https://doi.org/10.1016/j.actbio.2018.05.011

Ivens, I. A., Achanzar, W., Baumann, A., Brandli-Baiocco, A., Cavagnaro, J., Dempster, M., . . . Sims, J. (2015). PEGylated Biopharmaceuticals: Current Experience and Considerations for Nonclinical Development. *Toxicol Pathol, 43*(7), 959-983. doi:10.1177/0192623315591171

Jokerst, J. V., Lobovkina, T., Zare, R. N., & Gambhir, S. S. (2011). Nanoparticle PEGylation for imaging and therapy. *Nanomedicine (Lond), 6*(4), 715-728. doi:10.2217/nnm.11.19

Kanwal, U., Bukhari, N. I., Rana, N. F., Rehman, M., Hussain, K., Abbas, N., . . . Raza, A. (2019). Doxorubicin-loaded quaternary ammonium palmitoyl glycol chitosan polymeric nanoformulation: uptake by cells and organs. *Int J Nanomedicine, 14*, 1-15. doi:10.2147/ijn.S176868

Kaur, I. P., Bhandari, R., Bhandari, S., & Kakkar, V. (2008). Potential of solid lipid nanoparticles in brain targeting. *J Control Release, 127*(2), 97-109. doi:10.1016/j.jconrel.2007.12.018

Kelkar SS, Reineke TM. Theranostics: Combining Imaging and Therapy. Bioconjugate Chem 2011;22:1879-1903.

Kievit, F. M., & Zhang, M. (2011). Cancer nanotheranostics: improving imaging and therapy by targeted delivery across biological barriers. *Adv Mater, 23*(36), H217-247. doi:10.1002/adma.201102313

Kim, T. H., Lee, S., & Chen, X. (2013). Nanotheranostics for personalized medicine. *Expert review of molecular diagnostics, 13*(3), 257-269. doi:10.1586/erm.13.15

Knights-Mitchell, S. S., & Romanowski, M. (2018). Near-Infrared Activated Release of Doxorubicin from Plasmon Resonant Liposomes. *Nanotheranostics, 2*(4), 295-305. doi:10.7150/ntno.22544

Kolate, A., Baradia, D., Patil, S., Vhora, I., Kore, G., & Misra, A. (2014). PEG — A versatile conjugating ligand for drugs and drug delivery systems. *Journal of Controlled Release, 192*, 67-81. doi:https://doi.org/10.1016/j.jconrel.2014.06.046

Kuang, Y., Zhang, K., Cao, Y., Chen, X., Wang, K., Liu, M., & Pei, R. (2017). Hydrophobic IR-780 Dye Encapsulated in cRGD-Conjugated Solid Lipid Nanoparticles for NIR Imaging-Guided Photothermal Therapy. *ACS Appl Mater Interfaces, 9*(14), 12217-12226. doi:10.1021/acsami.6b16705

Lee DY, Li KC. Molecular Theranostics: a primer for the imaging professional. AJR Am J Roentgenol 2011;197:318-324.

Li, J., Cai, P., Shalviri, A., Henderson, J. T., He, C., Foltz, W. D., . . . Wu, X. Y. (2014). A Multifunctional Polymeric Nanotheranostic System Delivers Doxorubicin and Imaging Agents across the Blood–Brain Barrier Targeting Brain Metastases of Breast Cancer. *ACS Nano, 8*(10), 9925-9940. doi:10.1021/nn501069c

Lin, S. Y., Huang, R. Y., Liao, W. C., Chuang, C. C., & Chang, C. W. (2018). Multifunctional PEGylated Albumin/IR780/Iron Oxide Nanocomplexes for Cancer Photothermal Therapy and MR Imaging. *Nanotheranostics, 2*(2), 106-116. doi:10.7150/ntno.19379

Liu, G., Li, Y., Yang, L., Wei, Y., Wang, X., Wang, Z., & Tao, L. (2017). Cytotoxicity study of polyethylene glycol derivatives. *RSC Advances, 7*(30), 18252-18259. doi:10.1039/C7RA00861A

Luk, B. T., & Zhang, L. (2014). Current Advances in Polymer-Based Nanotheranostics for Cancer Treatment and Diagnosis. *ACS Applied Materials & Interfaces, 6*(24), 21859-21873. doi:10.1021/am5036225

Ma, X., Song, Q., & Gao, X. (2018). Reconstituted high-density lipoproteins: novel biomimetic nanocarriers for drug delivery. *Acta Pharm Sin B, 8*(1), 51-63. doi:10.1016/j.apsb.2017.11.006

Ma, Y., Tong, S., Bao, G., Gao, C., & Dai, Z. (2013). Indocyanine green loaded SPIO nanoparticles with phospholipid-PEG coating for dual-modal imaging and photothermal therapy. *Biomaterials, 34*(31), 7706-7714. doi:10.1016/j.biomaterials.2013.07.007

Miller, A. D. (2013). Lipid-Based Nanoparticles in Cancer Diagnosis and Therapy %J Journal of Drug Delivery. *2013*, 9. doi:10.1155/2013/165981

Mishra, P., Nayak, B., & Dey, R. K. (2016). PEGylation in anti-cancer therapy: An overview. *Asian Journal of Pharmaceutical Sciences, 11*(3), 337-348. doi:https://doi.org/10.1016/j.ajps.2015.08.011

Mishra, V., Bansal, K. K., Verma, A., Yadav, N., Thakur, S., Sudhakar, K., & Rosenholm, J. M. (2018). Solid Lipid Nanoparticles: Emerging Colloidal Nano Drug Delivery Systems. *Pharmaceutics, 10*(4). doi:10.3390/pharmaceutics10040191

Mooberry, L. K., Sabnis, N. A., Panchoo, M., Nagarajan, B., & Lacko, A. G. (2016). Targeting the SR-B1 Receptor as a Gateway for Cancer Therapy and Imaging. *Front Pharmacol, 7*, 466. doi:10.3389/fphar.2016.00466

Mulder, W. J., Strijkers, G. J., van Tilborg, G. A., Griffioen, A. W., & Nicolay, K. (2006). Lipid-based nanoparticles for contrast-enhanced MRI and molecular imaging. *NMR Biomed, 19*(1), 142-164. doi:10.1002/nbm.1011

Muthu, M. S., Leong, D. T., Mei, L., & Feng, S. S. (2014). Nanotheranostics - application and further development of nanomedicine strategies for advanced theranostics. *Theranostics, 4*(6), 660-677. doi:10.7150/thno.8698

Naseri, N., Valizadeh, H., & Zakeri-Milani, P. (2015). Solid Lipid Nanoparticles and Nanostructured Lipid Carriers: Structure, Preparation and Application. *Adv Pharm Bull, 5*(3), 305-313. doi:10.15171/apb.2015.043

Nayak, K. A. and Pal, D. (2010) Nanotechnology for Targeted Delivery in Cancer Therapeutics, Seemanta Institute of Pharmaceutical Sciences, Vol : 1 , Issue : 1.

Nehru, M. R. and Singh, P. O. (2008) Nanotechnology and Cancer Treatment , Asian J. Exp. Sci., Vol : 22 , No : 2 , 45 – 50.

Nie, S., Zhang, J., Martinez-Zaguilan, R., Sennoune, S., Hossen, M. N., Lichtenstein, A. H., . . . Wang, S. (2015). Detection of atherosclerotic lesions and intimal macrophages using CD36-targeted nanovesicles. *J Control Release, 220*(Pt A), 61-70. doi:10.1016/j.jconrel.2015.10.004

Palao-Suay, R., Martin-Saavedra, F. M., Rosa Aguilar, M., Escudero-Duch, C., Martin-Saldana, S., Parra-Ruiz, F. J., . . . San Roman, J. (2017). Photothermal and photodynamic activity of polymeric nanoparticles based on alpha-tocopheryl succinate-RAFT block copolymers conjugated to IR-780. *Acta Biomater, 57*, 70-84. doi:10.1016/j.actbio.2017.05.028

Raut, S., Mooberry, L., Sabnis, N., Garud, A., Dossou, A. S., & Lacko, A. (2018). Reconstituted HDL: Drug Delivery Platform for Overcoming Biological Barriers to Cancer Therapy. *Front Pharmacol, 9*, 1154. doi:10.3389/fphar.2018.01154

Seleci, M., Ag Seleci, D., Scheper, T., & Stahl, F. (2017). Theranostic Liposome-Nanoparticle Hybrids for Drug Delivery and Bioimaging. *Int J Mol Sci, 18*(7). doi:10.3390/ijms18071415

Sharon, P. E. , Ephrat, L. L. (2003) A Risky Business – Accessing Breast Cancer Risks , Science , 302 : 574 – 575

Singh, KK (2005) Nanotechnology in Cancer Detection and Treatment , Technology in Cancer Research and Treatment , 4 : 583 – 584

Sisay, B., Abrha, S., Yilma, Z., Assen, A., Molla, F., Tadese, E., Wondimu, A., Gebre-Samuel, N., Pattnaik, G. . (2014). CANCER NANOTHERANOSTICS: A NEW PARADIGM OF SIMULTANEOUS DIAGNOSIS AND THERAPY. *Journal of Drug Delivery and Therapeutics, 4(5)*, 79-86. doi: https://doi.org/10.22270/jddt.v4i5.967

Song, L., Able, S., Johnson, E., & Vallis, K. A. (2017). Accumulation of (111)In-Labelled EGF-Au-PEG Nanoparticles in EGFR-Positive Tumours is Enhanced by Coadministration of Targeting Ligand. *Nanotheranostics, 1*(3), 232-243. doi:10.7150/ntno.19952

Suk, J. S., Xu, Q., Kim, N., Hanes, J., & Ensign, L. M. (2016). PEGylation as a strategy for improving nanoparticle-based drug and gene delivery. *Adv Drug Deliv Rev, 99*(Pt A), 28-51. doi:10.1016/j.addr.2015.09.012

Sun, C., Wen, L., Zeng, J., Wang, Y., Sun, Q., Deng, L., . . . Li, Z. (2016). One-pot solventless preparation of PEGylated black phosphorus nanoparticles for photoacoustic imaging and photothermal therapy of cancer. *Biomaterials, 91*, 81-89. doi:10.1016/j.biomaterials.2016.03.022

Sumer, B. , Gao, J. (2008) Theranostic Nanomedicine for Cancer , Future Medicine , 3 (2) : 137 – 140 .

Tang, W. L., Tang, W. H., & Li, S. D. (2018). Cancer theranostic applications of lipid-based nanoparticles. *Drug Discov Today, 23*(5), 1159-1166. doi:10.1016/j.drudis.2018.04.007

Thaxton, C. S., Rink, J. S., Naha, P. C., & Cormode, D. P. (2016). Lipoproteins and lipoprotein mimetics for imaging and drug delivery. *Adv Drug Deliv Rev, 106*(Pt A), 116-131. doi:10.1016/j.addr.2016.04.020

Tripodo, G., Trapani, A., Torre, M. L., Giammona, G., Trapani, G., & Mandracchia, D. (2015). Hyaluronic acid and its derivatives in drug delivery and imaging: Recent advances and challenges. *Eur J Pharm Biopharm, 97*(Pt B), 400-416. doi:10.1016/j.ejpb.2015.03.032

Valetti, S., Mura, S., Stella, B., & Couvreur, P. (2013). Rational design for multifunctional non-liposomal lipid-based nanocarriers for cancer management: theory to practice. *J Nanobiotechnology, 11 Suppl 1*, S6. doi:10.1186/1477-3155-11-s1-s6

van Witteloostuijn, S. B., Pedersen, S. L., & Jensen, K. J. (2016). Half-Life Extension of Biopharmaceuticals using Chemical Methods: Alternatives to PEGylation. *11*(22), 2474-2495. doi:doi:10.1002/cmdc.201600374

Vllasaliu, D., Fowler, R., & Stolnik, S. (2014). PEGylated nanomedicines: recent progress and remaining concerns. *Expert Opinion on Drug Delivery, 11*(1), 139-154. doi:10.1517/17425247.2014.866651

Wang, J., Guo, F., Yu, M., Liu, L., Tan, F., Yan, R., & Li, N. (2016). Rapamycin/DiR loaded lipid-polyaniline nanoparticles for dual-modal imaging guided enhanced photothermal and antiangiogenic combination therapy. *J Control Release, 237*, 23-34. doi:10.1016/j.jconrel.2016.07.005

Wang, X. , Wang, Y. , Chen, Z. , Shin, M. D. (2009) Advances of Cancer Therapy by Nanotechnology , Cancer Res. Treat. , 41 (1) : 1 – 11.

Xing, H., Hwang, K., & Lu, Y. (2016). Recent Developments of Liposomes as Nanocarriers for Theranostic Applications. *Theranostics, 6*(9), 1336-1352. doi:10.7150/thno.15464

Xiong, F., Nirupama, S., Sirsi, S. R., Lacko, A., & Hoyt, K. (2017). Ultrasound-Stimulated Drug Delivery Using Therapeutic Reconstituted High-Density Lipoprotein Nanoparticles. *Nanotheranostics, 1*(4), 440-449. doi:10.7150/ntno.21905

Yang Y, Jing L, Li X, Lin L, Yue X, Dai Z. Hyaluronic Acid Conjugated Magnetic Prussian Blue@Quantum Dot Nanoparticles for Cancer Theranostics. Theranostics 2017; 7(2):466-481. doi:10.7150/thno.17411